Contents

Chapter 1: Introduction to COPD and Diet

Chronic Obstructive Pulmonary Disease (COPD) is a prevalent and potentially debilitating respiratory condition that affects millions of people worldwide. In this chapter, we will explore the fundamentals of COPD and its intricate relationship with diet. Understanding the impact of nutrition on COPD management is crucial for patients and caregivers seeking to improve quality of life and enhance overall well-being.

1.1 What is COPD?

COPD is a chronic lung disease characterized by impaired airflow, leading to difficulties in breathing. The two primary conditions associated with COPD are emphysema and chronic bronchitis, often coexisting in patients. Emphysema involves damage to the air sacs in the lungs, reducing their elasticity, while chronic bronchitis involves inflammation and narrowing of the airways, leading to increased mucus production. These conditions lead to persistent coughing, shortness of breath, wheezing, and fatigue, which progressively worsen over time.

1.2 The Importance of Diet in Managing COPD

While there is no cure for COPD, various strategies can help manage symptoms and slow disease progression. Among these, proper nutrition plays a significant role. A balanced diet provides essential nutrients to support the immune system, aid in respiratory function, and maintain overall health.

1.3 Consulting with a Healthcare Professional

Before making any significant dietary changes, individuals with COPD should consult with their healthcare provider or a registered dietitian. Each patient's nutritional needs are unique, depending on factors like age, weight, disease severity, and other existing health conditions. An expert can help tailor a personalized diet plan to address individual requirements effectively.

1.4 Key Nutrients in COPD Diet

Certain nutrients are particularly beneficial for COPD patients due to their positive impact on respiratory health and overall well-being. Let's explore some of these key nutrients and their significance:

Protein:

Protein is vital for maintaining and repairing body tissues, including the respiratory system. Adequate protein intake can help preserve respiratory muscle strength and support the immune system. Good sources of protein include lean meats, fish, poultry, legumes, and dairy products.

Antioxidants:

COPD is associated with increased oxidative stress, which can lead to further lung damage. Antioxidant-rich foods, such as fruits and vegetables (especially those rich in vitamin C and E), help neutralize harmful free radicals and reduce inflammation.

Omega-3 Fatty Acids:

Found in fatty fish (e.g., salmon, mackerel, and sardines), flaxseeds, and chia seeds, omega-3 fatty acids have anti-inflammatory properties that may benefit COPD patients by reducing inflammation in the lungs.

1.4.4 Fiber: A diet high in fiber promotes healthy digestion and can help prevent constipation, which may be exacerbated by certain COPD medications. Whole grains, fruits, vegetables, and legumes are excellent sources of dietary fiber.

Hydration and COPD

Staying adequately hydrated is essential for individuals with COPD. Proper hydration helps keep mucus thin and more manageable, reducing the likelihood of mucus plugs and easing breathing difficulties. It is recommended to drink sufficient water throughout the day, but fluid intake should be adjusted as per individual health needs and any existing conditions (e.g., heart disease, kidney problems).

In this chapter, we have introduced COPD as a chronic respiratory disease characterized by airflow obstruction, leading to various symptoms affecting breathing and overall lung function. We've emphasized the vital role of diet in managing COPD, and the significance of consulting with healthcare professionals to develop personalized nutrition plans.

The following chapters will delve deeper into nutritional guidelines, specific food recommendations, meal planning strategies, and lifestyle tips that can help COPD patients optimize their dietary habits for better respiratory health and an improved quality of life.

Chapter 2: Nutritional Guidelines for COPD Patient

In this chapter, we will explore essential nutritional guidelines that are crucial for managing Chronic Obstructive Pulmonary Disease (COPD). A balanced diet plays a pivotal role in supporting respiratory health, maintaining overall well-being, and potentially slowing the progression of the disease. Understanding the caloric needs, macronutrient balance, and the role of micronutrients in COPD management is vital for patients and caregivers seeking to optimize their dietary choices.

Caloric Needs and Energy Expenditure

COPD places an increased metabolic demand on the body, as the act of breathing requires more energy for individuals with impaired lung function. Therefore, COPD patients may have higher caloric needs than those without respiratory conditions. However, the caloric requirement varies from person to person based on factors like age, gender, weight, level of physical activity, and the severity of the disease.

It is essential for COPD patients to ensure that they consume enough calories to meet their energy expenditure while also avoiding excessive weight gain, which can further strain the respiratory system. A healthcare provider or registered dietitian can help determine the appropriate caloric intake for each individual.

Macronutrient Balance

(Carbohydrates, Proteins, Fats)

Balancing macronutrients in the diet is crucial for maintaining respiratory health and overall wellness. Each macronutrient serves specific functions in the body:

Carbohydrates:

Carbohydrates are the primary source of energy for the body. Complex carbohydrates, found in whole grains, fruits, and vegetables, are preferable over simple sugars. They provide sustained energy and a steady release of glucose, which is essential for individuals with COPD to manage their energy levels effectively.

Proteins:

Protein is essential for repairing body tissues, supporting the immune system, and maintaining muscle mass. Adequate protein intake is particularly crucial for COPD patients to preserve respiratory muscle strength, as breathing difficulties can lead to muscle wasting.

Fats:

Healthy fats, such as monounsaturated and polyunsaturated fats, are beneficial for COPD patients due to their anti-inflammatory properties. Sources of these fats include avocados, olive oil, nuts, and fatty fish. On the other hand, trans fats and saturated fats should be limited, as they can contribute to inflammation and worsen COPD symptoms.

Micronutrients and COPD

Micronutrients, including vitamins and minerals, are essential for various biochemical processes in the body. In COPD patients, certain micronutrients play a crucial role in supporting respiratory health and reducing inflammation. Some key micronutrients include:

Vitamin C:

An antioxidant that helps protect the lungs from oxidative damage caused by free radicals. Citrus fruits, strawberries, kiwis, and bell peppers are excellent sources of vitamin C.

Vitamin E:

Another antioxidant that supports lung health and helps counteract oxidative stress. Nuts, seeds, and vegetable oils are good sources of vitamin E.

Vitamin D:

Vital for maintaining bone health and a healthy immune system, vitamin D may also play a role in reducing COPD exacerbations. Fatty fish, fortified dairy products, and exposure to sunlight are sources of vitamin D.

Magnesium:

Helps relax the muscles, including the airway muscles, and may aid in reducing bronchial constriction. Leafy greens, nuts, seeds, and whole grains are magnesium-rich foods.

Zinc:

Supports the immune system and helps with wound healing. Zinc can be found in lean meats, seafood, nuts, and seeds.

Hydration and Fluid Intake

Staying well-hydrated is essential for COPD patients. Proper hydration helps keep mucus thin and more manageable, reducing the likelihood of mucus plugs and easing breathing difficulties. It is recommended to drink sufficient water throughout the day, but fluid intake should be adjusted as per individual health needs and any existing conditions (e.g., heart disease, kidney problems).

Chapter 2 has provided an overview of the nutritional guidelines for COPD patients. It emphasizes the importance of understanding individual caloric needs, balancing macronutrients, and ensuring adequate intake of essential micronutrients. By following these guidelines, COPD patients can optimize their nutritional intake to support respiratory health, enhance overall well-being, and potentially slow the progression of the disease. In the next chapter, we will delve into specific foods that are beneficial for COPD patients and those that should be limited or avoided.

Chapter 3: Foods to Emphasize in a COPD Diet

In this chapter, we will explore a variety of nutrient-dense foods that are particularly beneficial for individuals with Chronic Obstructive Pulmonary Disease (COPD). A well-balanced diet consisting of these foods can provide essential nutrients to support respiratory health, boost the immune system, and enhance overall well-being. Let's delve into the specific foods that should be emphasized in a COPD diet:

High-Fiber Foods

Fiber-rich foods are essential for maintaining digestive health and can be particularly helpful for COPD patients. Constipation is a common issue among those with COPD, often exacerbated by medications or reduced physical activity. Consuming enough fiber can promote regular bowel movements and prevent discomfort.

Excellent sources of dietary fiber include whole grains like oats, brown rice, quinoa, and whole wheat bread. Fruits such as apples, pears, berries, and bananas, as well as vegetables like broccoli, carrots, and sweet potatoes, are also rich in fiber.

Antioxidant-Rich Foods

COPD is associated with increased oxidative stress, which can lead to further lung damage. Antioxidants play a crucial role in neutralizing harmful free radicals, thereby reducing inflammation and protecting lung tissue.

Vitamin C and E are powerful antioxidants found in various fruits and vegetables. Citrus fruits like oranges, grapefruits, and lemons are excellent sources of vitamin C, while vitamin E can be found in nuts, seeds, and vegetable oils.

Omega-3 Fatty Acid Sources

Omega-3 fatty acids have anti-inflammatory properties that can be beneficial for COPD patients by reducing inflammation in the lungs. These essential fats are also known to support heart health and may have additional benefits for individuals with COPD.

Fatty fish such as salmon, mackerel, and sardines are excellent sources of omega-3 fatty acids. For those who prefer plant-based options, flaxseeds, chia seeds, and walnuts also provide a good supply of these beneficial fats.

Lean Proteins

Protein is essential for maintaining and repairing body tissues, including the respiratory system. COPD patients should prioritize lean sources of protein to avoid excess saturated fats, which can contribute to inflammation.

Skinless poultry, fish, legumes, tofu, and low-fat dairy products are excellent choices for lean protein. For those who consume meat, opting for lean cuts and cooking methods that use less added fat is recommended.

Vitamin D Source

Vitamin D is crucial for maintaining bone health and supporting the immune system. Some research suggests that vitamin D deficiency may be associated with more severe COPD symptoms and a higher risk of exacerbations.

While the body can produce vitamin D with exposure to sunlight, certain foods can also provide this essential nutrient. Fatty fish like salmon and mackerel, fortified dairy products (e.g., milk, yogurt), and fortified plant-based milk alternatives are good dietary sources of vitamin D.

Chapter 3 has highlighted essential foods to emphasize in a COPD diet. By incorporating high-fiber foods, antioxidant-rich fruits and vegetables, sources of omega-3 fatty acids, lean proteins, and vitamin D-rich foods, COPD patients can enhance their nutritional intake and support their respiratory health. A diet rich in these nutrient-dense foods can help reduce inflammation, strengthen the immune system, and potentially slow the progression of the disease. In the next chapter, we will discuss the importance of limiting or avoiding certain foods that may exacerbate COPD symptoms and negatively impact overall health.

Chapter 4: Foods to Avoid or Limit in a COPD Diet

In this chapter, we will explore specific foods that individuals with Chronic Obstructive Pulmonary Disease (COPD) should avoid or limit in their diet. Making informed choices about the foods we consume is crucial for managing COPD symptoms and promoting overall health. By understanding how certain foods can negatively impact respiratory function and exacerbate COPD symptoms, patients can make dietary adjustments to improve their quality of life.

Sodium and Its Impact on COPD

Excessive sodium intake can lead to fluid retention and increased blood pressure, potentially placing additional strain on the heart and lungs. For individuals with COPD, who may already experience breathing difficulties, the retention of fluids can make breathing even more challenging. Additionally, high sodium intake can lead to inflammation, which can worsen COPD symptoms.

Foods high in sodium include processed foods (e.g., packaged snacks, frozen meals, canned soups), fast foods, and certain condiments (e.g., soy sauce, ketchup). Instead, individuals with COPD should focus on using herbs and spices to flavor their meals and choose fresh, whole foods with lower sodium content.

Processed Foods and Trans Fats

Processed foods are typically high in unhealthy fats, including trans fats, which have been linked to increased inflammation and a higher risk of cardiovascular disease. For individuals with COPD, inflammation in the lungs can exacerbate symptoms and reduce respiratory function, making it important to limit inflammatory foods

Trans fats are commonly found in fried foods, baked goods (e.g., pastries, cookies, crackers), and some margarine products. Reading food labels can help identify products with trans fats, as they are often listed under "partially hydrogenated oils." Instead of processed foods, COPD patients should choose whole, nutrient-dense foods that are rich in vitamins, minerals, and healthy fats.

Excessive Caffeine and Alcohol

Caffeine and alcohol consumption can affect individuals with COPD in different ways.

Caffeine:

While moderate caffeine intake is generally safe for most people, excessive caffeine can lead to increased heart rate and potential anxiety, which may negatively impact breathing in COPD patients. Caffeine can also act as a diuretic, potentially contributing to dehydration

Limiting caffeine intake by moderating coffee, tea, and energy drink consumption can be beneficial for COPD patients. Opting for decaffeinated versions or herbal teas can still provide enjoyable beverage options.

4.3.2 Alcohol: Alcohol can interfere with the functioning of the respiratory system, particularly when consumed in excess. It can also interact with certain medications prescribed for COPD, potentially reducing their effectiveness

Individuals with COPD should consume alcohol in moderation or as advised by their healthcare provider, especially if they are taking medications that may interact with alcohol. Staying hydrated with water or other non-alcoholic beverages is crucial to maintain respiratory health

Gas-Inducing Foods

Certain foods can cause excess gas and bloating, which may lead to discomfort and worsen breathing difficulties in individuals with COPD.

While not everyone may experience the same reactions, it can be helpful to identify and limit gas-inducing foods.

Common gas-producing foods include beans, lentils, broccoli, cabbage, onions, and carbonated beverages. It is essential for COPD patients to monitor their individual tolerance to these foods and consider reducing or avoiding them if they cause discomfort.

Chapter 4 has discussed the importance of avoiding or limiting specific foods in a COPD diet. By reducing sodium intake, avoiding processed foods and trans fats, moderating caffeine and alcohol consumption, and identifying gas-inducing foods, individuals with COPD can improve their respiratory function and overall well-being. A well-balanced and mindful approach to dietary choices can complement COPD management and contribute to a better quality of life. In the next chapter, we will focus on meal planning strategies and offer practical tips for designing COPD-friendly meals and snacks that support respiratory health and overall nutritional needs.

Meal Planning for COPD Patients

In this chapter, we will explore meal planning strategies specifically tailored to individuals with Chronic Obstructive Pulmonary Disease (COPD). Proper meal planning is essential for managing respiratory health, supporting energy levels, and ensuring adequate nutrient intake. By designing COPD-friendly meals and snacks, patients can optimize their dietary choices and enhance their overall well-being.

Balancing Nutrient Intake

A well-balanced diet is crucial for individuals with COPD to ensure they receive all the essential nutrients needed for optimal respiratory function and overall health. This includes consuming a mix of carbohydrates, proteins, and healthy fats in appropriate proportions.

COPD patients should aim to include a variety of nutrient-dense foods in their meals. Whole grains, such as brown rice, quinoa, and oats, provide valuable carbohydrates for sustained energy. Lean proteins, like poultry, fish, legumes, and tofu, aid in maintaining muscle mass and supporting the immune system. Healthy fats, found in foods like avocados, nuts, seeds, and fatty fish, have anti-inflammatory properties that can benefit COPD patients.

Smaller, Frequent Meals vs. Larger Meals

COPD patients often experience shortness of breath and fatigue, which can make eating larger meals challenging. Consuming smaller, more frequent meals throughout the day can be a practical approach to meet nutrient needs while minimizing the discomfort associated with overeating.

Dividing daily caloric intake into five or six smaller meals and snacks can help prevent feelings of fullness or bloating, making it easier to breathe comfortably. This meal pattern also helps maintain steady energy levels and may aid in preventing rapid spikes and drops in blood sugar.

Portable and Easy-to-Prepare Meals

For individuals with COPD who may have limited energy or find cooking physically taxing, portable and easy-to-prepare meals are a practical solution. Having readily available, nutritious options can prevent reliance on processed or unhealthy convenience foods.

Some examples of portable and easy-to-prepare meals include whole-grain sandwiches with lean protein and vegetables, pre-cut fruit and vegetable packs, yogurt cups, and homemade trail mix with nuts and dried fruits.

Snack Options for COPD Patients

Healthy snacks can provide a source of energy and nutrients between meals, helping to maintain stable blood sugar levels and prevent excessive hunger. COPD patients should choose snacks that are easy to digest and do not cause discomfort or excess gas.

Some nutritious snack options for COPD patients include whole-grain crackers with hummus, Greek yogurt with fresh berries, sliced apples with nut butter, or a handful of mixed nuts and seeds.

Fluid Intake and Hydratio

Staying well-hydrated is essential for COPD patients to keep mucus thin and easier to manage. However, drinking large amounts of fluids during meals can lead to feeling overly full and increase the discomfort of shortness of breath.

To balance hydration and comfort, it is advisable for COPD patients to focus on consuming fluids between meals rather than during meals. Sipping water, herbal teas, or other non-caffeinated beverages throughout the day can help maintain adequate hydration without causing discomfort.

Monitoring and Recording Meals

Keeping a food journal or using a mobile app to track meals and snacks can be beneficial for COPD patients. This practice allows individuals to monitor their nutrient intake, identify patterns or triggers for symptoms, and make adjustments to their diet as needed.

By recording meals and symptoms, COPD patients can work with their healthcare provider or a registered dietitian to make targeted dietary changes that support their specific health goals.

Chapter 5 has explored meal planning strategies tailored to individuals with COPD. Balancing nutrient intake, choosing smaller, frequent meals, opting for portable and easy-to-prepare options, selecting nutritious snacks, and monitoring fluid intake are key considerations for COPD-friendly meal planning. By incorporating these strategies, COPD patients can maintain optimal respiratory health, manage energy levels, and enjoy a diverse and satisfying diet. In the next chapter, we will discuss COPD-friendly recipes that showcase delicious and nutrient-rich meals suitable for individuals with respiratory conditions.

Chapter 6: COPD-Friendly Recipes

In this chapter, we will explore a collection of delicious and nutrient-rich recipes tailored to individuals with Chronic Obstructive Pulmonary Disease (COPD). These recipes are designed to support respiratory health, provide essential nutrients, and cater to the specific dietary needs of COPD patients. By incorporating these COPD-friendly recipes into their meal planning, individuals can enjoy a diverse and satisfying diet that enhances overall well-being.

Breakfast Ideas

Breakfast is an important meal that sets the tone for the day and provides essential nutrients and energy. For COPD patients, a balanced breakfast can help maintain energy levels, support respiratory function, and promote overall health.

A. Veggie Omelet:

Ingredients:

- 2 large eggs

- 1/4 cup diced bell peppers

- 1/4 cup diced onions

- 1/4 cup diced tomatoes

- 1/4 cup chopped spinach

- 1 tablespoon olive oil

- Salt and pepper to taste

Instructions:

1. In a bowl, whisk the eggs until well beaten. Add salt and pepper to taste.

2. In a non-stick skillet, heat the olive oil over medium heat.

3. Add the diced bell peppers, onions, tomatoes, and spinach to the skillet. Cook until the vegetables are tender.

4. Pour the beaten eggs over the cooked vegetables in the skillet. Cook until the eggs are set and the bottom is lightly browned.

5. Fold the omelet in half and cook for another minute until fully cooked.

B. Overnight Oats:

Ingredients:

- 1/2 cup rolled oats

- 1/2 cup milk or plant-based milk

- 1/2 cup Greek yogurt

- 1 tablespoon chia seeds

- 1 tablespoon honey or maple syrup

- Fresh berries for topping

Instructions:

1. In a mason jar or container with a lid, combine the rolled oats, milk, Greek yogurt, chia seeds, and honey or maple syrup.

2. Stir well to mix all the ingredients thoroughly.

3. Cover the jar or container and refrigerate overnight.

4. In the morning, top the overnight oats with fresh berries before serving.

Lunch and Dinner Recipe

Lunch and dinner are opportunities to enjoy satisfying and nourishing meals that support respiratory health and overall well-being

A. Grilled Salmon with Quinoa and Roasted Vegetables:

Ingredients:

- 1 salmon fillet

- 1 cup cooked quinoa

- Assorted vegetables (e.g., broccoli, bell peppers, zucchini)

- 1 tablespoon olive oil

- Lemon wedges for serving

- Fresh dill for garnish

- Salt and pepper to taste

Instructions:

1. Preheat the grill or oven to medium-high heat.

2. Season the salmon fillet with salt and pepper and drizzle with olive oil.

3. Grill or bake the salmon until fully cooked and flaky.

4. While the salmon is cooking, toss the vegetables in olive oil, salt, and pepper. Roast them in the oven until tender.

5. Serve the grilled salmon over a bed of cooked quinoa, with roasted vegetables on the side.

6. Garnish with fresh dill and serve with lemon wedges.

B. Tomato Basil Pasta with Shrimp:

Ingredients:

- 1 cup whole-grain pasta

- 1 cup cherry tomatoes, halved

- 1/2 cup fresh basil leaves, chopped

- 1/4 cup grated Parmesan cheese

- 1 tablespoon olive oil

- 1 clove garlic, minced

- 1/2 pound shrimp, peeled and deveined

- Salt and pepper to taste

Instructions:

1. Cook the whole-grain pasta according to the package instructions. Drain and set aside.

2. In a large skillet, heat the olive oil over medium heat. Add the minced garlic and cook for about 1 minute until fragrant.

3. Add the shrimp to the skillet and cook until they turn pink and are fully cooked.

4. Toss the cooked pasta, cherry tomatoes, and chopped basil in the skillet with the shrimp.

5. Season with salt and pepper to taste and stir well to combine all the ingredients.

6. Sprinkle grated Parmesan cheese over the pasta before serving.

Soups and Stews

Soups and stews are comforting and nourishing options that can be packed with nutrients to support respiratory health.

A. Chicken and Vegetable Soup:

Ingredients:

- 1 tablespoon olive oil

- 1 onion, diced

- 2 carrots, peeled and diced

- 2 celery stalks, diced

- 2 garlic cloves, minced

- 6 cups low-sodium chicken broth

- 2 cups cooked and shredded chicken breast

- 1 cup diced tomatoes (canned or fresh)

- 1 cup chopped spinach

- 1 teaspoon dried thyme

- Salt and pepper to taste

Instructions:

1. In a large pot, heat the olive oil over medium heat. Add the diced onion, carrots, and celery. Cook until the vegetables are softened.

2. Add the minced garlic and cook for another minute until fragrant.

3. Pour in the chicken broth and bring it to a simmer.

4. Add the shredded chicken, diced tomatoes, chopped spinach, and dried thyme to the pot.

5. Let the soup simmer for about 15 minutes to allow the flavors to meld.

6. Season with salt and pepper to taste before serving.

B. Lentil and Vegetable Stew:

Ingredients:

- 1 tablespoon olive oil

- 1 onion, diced

- 2 carrots, peeled and diced

- 2 celery stalks, diced

- 2 garlic cloves, minced

- 1 cup dried lentils, rinsed and drained

- 4 cups vegetable broth

- 1 cup diced potatoes

- 1 cup diced tomatoes (canned or fresh)

- 1 teaspoon ground cumin

- 1/2 teaspoon paprika

- Salt and pepper to taste

Instructions:

1. In a large pot, heat the olive oil over medium heat. Add the diced onion, carrots, and celery. Cook until the vegetables are softened.

2. Add the minced garlic and cook for another minute until fragrant.

3. Stir in the dried lentils, vegetable broth, diced potatoes, diced tomatoes, ground cumin, and paprika.

4. Bring the stew to a boil, then reduce the heat and let it simmer for about 20-25 minutes until the lentils and potatoes are tender.

5. Season with salt and pepper to taste before serving.

Snack and Smoothie Recipes

Snacks and smoothies can be nutritious and enjoyable ways to maintain energy levels and support respiratory health between meals.

A. Nut Butter and Banana Rice Cakes:

Ingredients:

- 2 rice cakes

- 2 tablespoons nut butter (peanut butter, almond butter, etc.)

- 1 small banana, sliced

Instructions:

1. Spread nut butter evenly on each rice cake.

2. Arrange the sliced banana on top of the nut butter.

3. Sandwich the rice cakes together, nut butter and banana sides facing each other.

4. Enjoy as a portable and nutritious snack.

B. Green Smoothie:

Ingredients:

- 1 cup fresh spinach leaves

- 1/2 cup diced pineapple

- 1/2 cup diced cucumber

- 1 small banana

- 1 cup

 coconut water or plant-based milk

- Ice cubes (optional)

Instructions:

1. In a blender, combine fresh spinach, diced pineapple, diced cucumber, and a small banana.

2. Add coconut water or plant-based milk to the blender.

3. Blend all the ingredients until smooth and creamy.

4. Add ice cubes if desired and blend again.

5. Pour the green smoothie into a glass and enjoy a refreshing and nutrient-packed drink.

Chapter 6 has presented a selection of COPD-friendly recipes that cater to the specific dietary needs of individuals with Chronic Obstructive Pulmonary Disease. These delicious and nutrient-rich recipes showcase a variety of breakfast ideas, lunch and dinner options, soups and stews, and snacks and smoothies. By incorporating these recipes into their meal planning, COPD patients can enjoy satisfying and nourishing meals that support respiratory health and overall well-being. In the next chapter, we will discuss eating strategies to cope with shortness of breath while eating, tips for easier swallowing, and strategies for managing weight and hydration in COPD patients.

Chapter 7: Eating Strategies for COPD Symptom Management

In this chapter, we will explore various eating strategies tailored to individuals with Chronic Obstructive Pulmonary Disease (COPD). COPD patients often experience symptoms like shortness of breath and difficulty swallowing, which can impact their ability to eat comfortably. By implementing specific eating strategies, individuals can manage these symptoms effectively, ensure adequate nutrient intake, and enhance their overall dining experience.

Coping with Shortness of Breath While Eating

Shortness of breath is a common symptom experienced by individuals with COPD, and it can be particularly challenging during mealtime. The act of eating and breathing simultaneously can cause discomfort and make eating feel more exhausting. However, there are strategies to cope with shortness of breath while eating:

A. Paced Eating: Take your time when eating and avoid rushing through meals. Eating slowly and mindfully can help reduce the strain on your respiratory system and allow you to enjoy your food more fully.

B. Breathing Techniques: Practice deep breathing exercises before and during meals. Inhale deeply through your nose and exhale slowly through your mouth. This can help you stay relaxed and ease shortness of breath while eating.

C. Small Bites: Take smaller, more manageable bites of food to reduce the need for prolonged chewing and make swallowing easier. Cutting food into smaller pieces can also be helpful.

D. Upright Position: Sit in an upright position while eating to promote better lung expansion and ease breathing. Avoid slouching or lying down during meals.

E. Rest Between Bites: Take short breaks between bites to catch your breath and avoid feeling overwhelmed while eating.

Tips for Easier Swallowing

In COPD, swallowing difficulties can arise due to weakened muscles or the feeling of breathlessness. Proper swallowing techniques can facilitate the process and minimize discomfort:

A. Stay Hydrated: Drink sufficient water between bites to help moisten the food and make swallowing easier. Adequate hydration can also prevent dry mouth, a common issue for COPD patients.

B. Chew Thoroughly: Take the time to chew your food thoroughly to break it down into smaller pieces before swallowing. This can reduce the effort required during the swallowing process.

C. Avoid Distractions: Focus on your meal and avoid distractions like watching TV or engaging in intense conversations. Concentrating on your food can help you pay attention to swallowing and prevent choking.

D. Modify Food Consistency: If swallowing is challenging, consider modifying the consistency of your food. Soft or pureed foods may be easier to swallow than harder or crunchy textures.

E. Consider Liquid Supplements: If swallowing solid foods becomes too difficult, liquid nutritional supplements can provide essential nutrients and calories.

7.3 Eating fo Weight Management

Maintaining a healthy weight is important for individuals with COPD, as being underweight or overweight can both pose challenges. Here are some tips for eating to manage weight:

A. Underweight COPD Patients:

   - Focus on nutrient-dense foods that provide a high number of calories in smaller portions.

   - Incorporate healthy fats, such as avocados, nuts, and olive oil, to increase caloric intake.

   - Eat frequent, smaller meals throughout the day to avoid feeling overly full.

B. Overweight COPD Patients:

   - Choose nutrient-dense, lower-calorie foods to support respiratory health while managing weight.

   - Practice portion control to avoid overeating.

- Engage in regular physical activity within your capabilities to promote weight management.

7.4 Staying Hydrated and Managing Mucus

Staying hydrated is crucial for individuals with COPD, as proper hydration helps keep mucus thin and more manageable, reducing the likelihood of mucus plugs and easing breathing difficulties. Here are some tips for staying hydrated and managing mucus:

A. Monitor Fluid Intake: Keep track of your daily fluid intake to ensure you are drinking enough water. Aim for at least eight 8-ounce glasses of water per day, but adjust this amount based on your individual needs and any medical restrictions.

B. Choose Hydrating Foods: Consume foods with high water content, such as fruits (e.g., watermelon, oranges) and vegetables (e.g., cucumbers, tomatoes), to supplement your fluid intake.

C. Use Humidifiers: Consider using a humidifier at home, especially during dry or cold weather, to help keep the air moist and ease breathing.

D. Avoid Dehydrating Substances: Limit your intake of dehydrating substances like caffeine and alcohol, as they can contribute to fluid loss.

7.5 Supplementation for COPD Patients

While a balanced diet should be the primary source of nutrients for COPD patients, certain individuals may benefit from dietary supplements to address specific deficiencies or support respiratory health. However, it's essential to consult with a healthcare provider or a registered dietitian before starting any supplements. Some supplements that may be considered for COPD patients include:

A. Omega-3 Fatty Acids: Fish oil supplements can provide additional anti-inflammatory benefits, supporting lung health for individuals with COPD.

B. Vitamin D: Supplements may be recommended for those with vitamin D deficiencies, as this nutrient is vital for immune function and respiratory health.

C. Probiotics: Probiotic supplements can help promote gut health and support overall immune function.

Chapter 7 has provided valuable eating strategies for managing COPD symptoms and supporting respiratory health. By coping with shortness of breath while eating, employing tips for easier swallowing, eating for weight management, staying hydrated, and considering appropriate supplementation, individuals with COPD can optimize their dietary habits to enhance overall well-being. In the next chapter, we will discuss lifestyle tips, including smoking cessation, pulmonary rehabilitation, exercise, stress management, and sleep hygiene, which can complement diet in improving COPD management and quality of life.

Introduction to the Zone Diet

The Zone Diet is a popular eating plan that focuses on balancing macronutrient ratios to promote weight loss and overall health. Developed by Dr. Barry Sears, a biochemist and researcher, the Zone Diet emphasizes the importance of maintaining a specific ratio of carbohydrates, proteins, and fats in each meal.

Brief explanation of the Zone Diet's principles

The Zone Diet is based on the concept that the body functions optimally when maintained within a specific hormonal "zone." By carefully controlling the macronutrient composition of meals, the diet aims to keep insulin levels stable and promote the production of anti-inflammatory compounds.

Emphasis on balanced macronutrient ratios

Unlike many other popular diets that restrict certain food groups or drastically reduce caloric intake, the Zone Diet focuses on creating a balance among macronutrients. The ideal ratio recommended in the Zone Diet is 40% carbohydrates, 30% protein, and 30% fat.

This balance is designed to provide a steady release of energy throughout the day, control hunger, and stabilize blood sugar levels. The macronutrient ratio is thought to regulate the production of insulin, which plays a crucial role in fat storage and metabolism.

By following the Zone Diet, individuals aim to achieve a state of hormonal balance that can lead to weight loss, improved body composition, enhanced athletic performance, and increased overall well-being.

The Zone Diet is not just about the quantity of food but also the quality. It encourages the consumption of whole, unprocessed foods such as lean proteins, fruits, vegetables, and healthy fats while minimizing refined carbohydrates, sugars, and processed foods.

In conclusion, the Zone Diet offers a unique approach to weight loss and health by focusing on maintaining a balanced macronutrient ratio. By carefully selecting and portioning out the right combination of carbohydrates, proteins, and fats, followers of the Zone Diet aim to achieve hormonal balance and optimize their overall well-being.

Understanding the Macronutrient Balance

A. Definition of macronutrients (carbohydrates, proteins, fats)

Macronutrients are the three main components of our diet that provide energy and are required in larger quantities by the body. They include carbohydrates, proteins, and fats.

Carbohydrates: Carbohydrates are the body's primary source of energy. They are found in foods like grains, fruits, vegetables, and legumes. Carbohydrates can be classified into simple (such as sugars) and complex (such as starches and fiber). They play a vital role in fueling the brain, muscles, and other bodily functions.

Proteins: Proteins are essential for the growth, repair, and maintenance of tissues in the body. They are made up of amino acids and can be found in sources like meat, poultry, fish, eggs, dairy products, legumes, and nuts. Proteins also contribute to the production of enzymes, hormones, and antibodies.

Fats: Fats are a concentrated source of energy and are involved in various bodily functions. They are categorized into saturated fats (found in animal products and some plant oils), unsaturated fats (found in nuts, seeds, and vegetable oils), and trans fats (found in processed and fried foods). Fats are important for hormone production, nutrient absorption, insulation, and protecting organs.

The optimal ratio of macronutrients in the Zone Diet (40:30:30)

The Zone Diet recommends a specific macronutrient ratio of 40% carbohydrates, 30% protein, and 30% fat. This balance is intended to control insulin levels and promote hormonal balance, which can lead to weight loss, improved body composition, and enhanced overall health.

Carbohydrates: The Zone Diet emphasizes the consumption of low glycemic carbohydrates, which have a slower and more sustained impact on blood sugar levels. Examples include whole grains, fruits, and vegetables. By focusing on these sources, the diet aims to avoid spikes and crashes in blood sugar, reducing hunger and maintaining energy levels.

Proteins: The Zone Diet encourages the inclusion of lean proteins such as chicken, fish, tofu, and legumes. Proteins help regulate appetite, promote muscle growth and repair, and provide a steady release of amino acids for various bodily functions. They also have a lower impact on insulin levels compared to carbohydrates.

Fats: The Zone Diet advocates for the consumption of healthy fats like olive oil, avocados, nuts, and seeds. These fats provide essential fatty acids, support brain function, and aid in nutrient absorption. The inclusion of fats in the diet also helps promote satiety and stabilize blood sugar levels.

C. Importance of maintaining balanced meals

Maintaining balanced meals is a key principle of the Zone Diet. This involves incorporating all three macronutrients in each meal to achieve the desired ratio. Here are some reasons why balanced meals are important:

Steady energy levels: Balanced meals that include carbohydrates, proteins, and fats provide a steady release of energy throughout the day. This helps prevent energy crashes and keeps you feeling more satisfied and energized.

Blood sugar control: Balanced meals can help regulate blood sugar levels by avoiding sudden spikes and drops. This is particularly beneficial for individuals with conditions such as diabetes or insulin resistance.

Appetite control: The combination of protein, carbohydrates, and fats in balanced meals helps promote satiety and control hunger. This can reduce the likelihood of overeating and snacking on unhealthy foods between meals.

Nutrient absorption: Consuming a variety of macronutrients in balanced meals enhances the absorption of essential vitamins and minerals. Certain nutrients require the presence of specific macronutrients for optimal absorption in the body.

Hormonal balance: Maintaining a balanced macronutrient ratio can help regulate insulin levels, which plays a significant role in fat storage and metabolism. By achieving hormonal balance, the Zone Diet aims to promote weight loss and overall health.

In summary, understanding the macronutrient balance is essential in following the Zone Diet. The recommended ratio of 40% carbohydrates, 30% protein, and 30% fat aims to promote hormonal balance and overall well-being. By incorporating all three macronutrients in balanced meals, individuals can experience steady energy levels, improved blood sugar control, appetite regulation, enhanced nutrient absorption, and hormonal balance.

The Zone Diet: A Complete Overview

The Zone Diet has been popular for several decades.

It encourages followers to eat a certain amount of protein, carbs and fat at every meal in order to reduce inflammation in the body, among other health benefits.

However, critics have targeted some of its health claims.

This article provides a detailed overview of the Zone Diet, including how to follow it, its benefits and disadvantages.

BOTTOM LINE: The Zone diet focuses on eating a specific ratio of macronutrients to combat inflammation. Though the eating pattern may be linked to several benefits, the proponents of the diet also make many strong and unfounded health claims around its efficacy.

What is the Zone Diet?

The Zone Diet instructs its followers to stick to eating a specific ratio of 40% carbs, 30% protein and 30% fat.

As part of the diet, carbs should have a low glycemic index, which means they provide a slow release of sugar into the blood to keep you fuller for longer. Protein should be lean and fat should be mostly monounsaturated.

The Zone Diet was developed more than 30 years ago by Dr. Barry Sears, an American biochemist. His best-selling book The Zone was published in 1995.

Dr. Sears developed this diet after losing family members to early deaths from heart attacks, and felt that he was at risk unless he found a way to fight it.

The Zone Diet claims to reduce the inflammation in your body. Dr. Sears proposed inflammation was the reason people gain weight, become sick and age faster.

Proponents of the diet claim that once you reduce inflammation, you will lose fat at the fastest rate possible, slow down aging, reduce your risk of chronic disease and improve your performance.

SUMMARY:

The Zone Diet follows a specific ratio of 40% carbs, 30% protein and 30% fat. It was created by Dr. Barry Sears more than 30 years ago.

How do you follow the Zone Diet?

The Zone Diet has no specific phases and is designed to be followed for a lifetime.

There are two ways to follow the Zone Diet: the hand-eye method, or using Zone food blocks.

Most people start with the hand-eye method and progress to using Zone food blocks later, since it is more advanced. You can switch between both methods whenever you feel like, since they each have their own benefits.

The hand-eye method

The hand-eye method is the easiest way to start the Zone Diet.

As the name suggests, your hand and eye are the only tools you need to get started, although wearing a watch is also recommended to keep an eye on when to eat.

In this method, your hand takes on several uses. You use it to determine your portion sizes. Your five fingers remind you to eat five times a day and never go without food for five hours.

Meanwhile, you use your eye to estimate portions on your plate. To design a Zone-friendly plate, you need to first divide your plate into thirds.

• One-third lean protein: One-third of your plate should have a source of lean protein, roughly the size and thickness of your palm.

• Two-thirds carbs: Two-thirds of your plate should be filled with carbs with a low glycemic index.

• A little fat: Add a dash of monounsaturated fat to your plate, such as olive oil, avocado or almonds.

The hand-eye method is designed to be a simple way for a beginner to follow the Zone Diet.

It is also flexible and allows you to eat out at restaurants while on the Zone Diet, by using your hand and eyes as tools to choose options that fit Zone recommendations.

You can learn more about eating out on this diet here.

The Zone food block method

Zone food blocks allow you to personalize the Zone Diet to your body by calculating how many grams of protein, carbs and fat you can have per day.

The number of Zone blocks you should eat per day depends on your weight, height, waist and hip measurements. You can calculate your number here.

The average male eats 14 Zone blocks per day, while the average female eats 11 Zone blocks per day.

A main meal such as breakfast, lunch or dinner contains three to five Zone blocks, while a snack always contains one Zone block.

Each Zone block is made of a protein block, a fat block and a carb block.

• Protein block: Contains 7 grams of protein.

• Carb block: Contains 9 grams of carbs.

• Fat block: Contains 1.5 grams of fat.

Here is a detailed guide with different options and how much of each food option is needed to make a protein block, carb block or fat block.

SUMMARY:

You can choose to follow the Zone Diet with either the hand-eye method or the Zone food block method.

What foods can you eat on the Zone Diet?

A lot of the favorable Zone Diet food choices are similar to those of the Mediterranean Diet, which is one of the healthiest diets on the planet.

In fact, the creator of the Zone Diet has recently released a new book called The Mediterranean Zone, in which he covers the similarities and benefits of the two diets.

Protein

Protein options in the Zone Diet should be lean. Good options include:

• Lean beef, pork, lamb, veal and game

• Skinless chicken and turkey breast

• Fish and shellfish

• Vegetarian protein, tofu, other soy products

• Egg whites

• Low-fat cheeses

• Low-fat milk and yogurt

Fat

The Zone Diet encourages choosing a type of monounsaturated fat. Good options include:

• Avocados

• Nuts, such as macadamia, peanuts, cashews, almonds or pistachios

• Peanut butter

• Tahini

• Oils such as canola oil, sesame oil, peanut oil and olive oil

Carbs

The Zone Diet encourages its followers to choose vegetables with a low glycemic index and a little fruit.

Good options include:

- Fruit such as berries, apples, oranges, plums and more

- Vegetables such as cucumbers, peppers, spinach, tomatoes, mushrooms, yellow squash, chickpeas and more

- Grains, such as oatmeal and barley

SUMMARY:

Similar to the Mediterranean Diet, Zone Diet food options include lean protein, carbs with a low glycemic index and healthy fats.

What can't you eat on the Zone Diet?

Nothing is strictly banned on the Zone Diet. However, certain food choices are considered unfavorable because they promote inflammation.

- High-sugar fruits: Such as bananas, grapes, raisins, dried fruits and mangoes.

- High-sugar or starchy vegetables: Like peas, corn, carrots and potatoes.

- Refined and processed carbs: Bread, bagels, pasta, noodles and other white-flour products.

- Other processed foods: Including breakfast cereals and muffins.

- Foods with added sugar: Such as candy, cakes and cookies.

- Soft drinks: Neither sugar-sweetened nor sugar-free drinks are recommended.

- Coffee and tea: Keep these to a minimum, since water is the beverage of choice.

SUMMARY:

No food is banned on the Zone Diet, but foods that are not encouraged include those that are high in sugar and starch, are processed, or have refined carbs or added sugar. Water is the recommended beverage.

Sample food block meal plan for men

Here is a sample block meal plan with 14 food blocks, for the average man.

Breakfast (4 food blocks): Scrambled eggs with turkey bacon, vegetables and fruit.

- 2 eggs, scrambled

- 3 strips turkey bacon

- 1 ounce of low-fat cheese

- 1 apple

- 3 1/2 cups (630 grams) of spinach, cooked

- 1 cup (156 grams) mushrooms, boiled

- 1/4 cup (53 grams) onions, boiled

- 1 1/3 teaspoons (6.6 ml) olive oil

Lunch (4 food blocks): Grilled chicken and egg salad with fruit.

- 3 ounces (84 grams) grilled chicken, skinless

- 1 hard-boiled egg

- Up to 2 heads of iceberg lettuce

- 1 cup (70 grams) raw mushrooms

- 1 cup (104 grams) raw cucumber, sliced

- 1 red bell pepper, sliced

- 2 tablespoons avocado

- 1/2 teaspoon walnuts

- 1 teaspoon (5 ml) vinegar dressing

- 2 plums

Mid-Afternoon Snack (1 food block): Boiled egg, nuts and fruit.

- 1 hard-boiled egg

- 3 almonds

- 1/2 apple

Dinner (4 food blocks): Grilled salmon, lettuce and sweet potatoes.

- 6 ounces (170 grams) salmon, grilled

- 1 cup (200 grams) of sweet potatoes, baked

- Up to 1 head of iceberg lettuce

- 1/4 cup (37 grams) tomato, raw

- 1 cup (104 grams) raw cucumber, sliced

- 2 tablespoons avocado

- 2/3 teaspoon (3.3 ml) olive oil

Pre-Bedtime Snack (1 food block): Cottage cheese, nuts and fruit.

- 1/4 cup (56 grams) cottage cheese

- 6 peanuts

- 1/2 orange

SUMMARY:

The Zone Diet meal plans break food portions into food blocks, which give you the diet's proportions of macronutrients throughout the day.

Sample food block meal plan for women

Here is a sample block meal plan for the average female, with 11 food blocks.

Breakfast (3 food blocks): Scrambled eggs with turkey bacon and fruit.

- 2 eggs, scrambled

- 3 strips turkey bacon

- 1/2 apple

- 1 cup (156 grams) mushrooms, boiled

- 3 1/2 cups (630 grams) spinach, cooked

- 1 teaspoon (5 ml) olive oil

Lunch (3 food blocks): Grilled chicken and egg salad with fruit.

- 2 ounces (57 grams) grilled chicken, skinless

- 1 hard-boiled egg

- Up to 2 heads of iceberg lettuce

- 1 cup (70 grams) raw mushrooms

- 1 cup (104 grams) raw cucumber, sliced

- 1 sliced red pepper

- 2 tablespoons avocado

- 1 teaspoon (5 ml) vinegar dressing

- 1 plum

Mid-Afternoon Snack (1 food block): Boiled egg, nuts and fruit.

- 1 hard-boiled egg

- 3 almonds

- 1/2 apple

Dinner (3 food blocks): Grilled salmon, lettuce and sweet potatoes.

- 4 oz (113 grams) salmon, grilled

- 2/3 cup (67 grams) of sweet potatoes, baked

- Up to 1 head of iceberg lettuce

- 1/4 cup (37 grams) raw tomato

- 1 cup (104 grams) raw cucumber, sliced

- 2 tablespoons avocado

- 1/3 teaspoon (3.3 ml) olive oil

Pre-Bedtime Snack (1 food block): Cottage cheese, nuts and fruit.

- 1/4 cup (56 grams) cottage cheese

- 6 peanuts

- 1/2 orange

SUMMARY:

A sample meal plan for women is similar to the plan for men, but has 11 food blocks instead of 14.

How does the Zone Diet work?

The Zone Diet claims to optimize your hormones to allow your body to enter a state called "the Zone." This is where your body is optimized to control inflammation from your diet.

The purported benefits of being in "the Zone" are:

- Losing extra body fat as fast as possible

- Maintaining wellness into older age

- Slowing down the rate of aging

• Performing better and thinking faster

Dr. Sears recommends testing three blood values to determine whether you are in "the Zone."

TG/HDL ratio

This is the ratio of "bad" fats known as triglycerides to "good" HDL cholesterol in your blood. A lower value means you have more good cholesterol, which is healthier.

The Zone Diet recommends less than 1 as a good value, which is low. A high number for your TG/HDL ratio increases your risk of heart disease (1Trusted Source).

Your ratio for TG/HDL must be tested by a health care professional, such as your doctor.

AA/EPA ratio

This is the ratio of omega-6 to omega-3 fats in your body. A lower value means you have more omega-3 fat in your blood, which is anti-inflammatory.

The Zone Diet recommends a value between 1.5–3, which is low. A high number for your AA/EPA ratio is linked with a higher risk of depression, obesity and other chronic diseases.

You can test your ratio for AA/EPA at home with a kit purchased on the Zone Diet website.

HbA1c, also known as glycated hemoglobin

This is a marker of your average blood sugar levels over the preceding three months. A lower value means you have less sugar in your blood.

The Zone Diet recommends a value of less than 5%, which is low. A higher HbA1c is linked to a higher risk of diabetes.

Your HbA1c must be tested by a health care professional, such as your doctor.

Supplements recommended

The Zone Diet recommends that you take omega-3 supplements, such as fish oil, to maximize health benefits. They decrease the "bad" LDL cholesterol in your body, and may reduce your risk of other chronic health diseases.

The Zone Diet also recommends taking polyphenol supplements, which are molecules found in plants that have antioxidant properties.

The evidence behind polyphenols is mixed and although they may provide health benefits such as reducing the risk of heart disease, they also have risks such as decreasing your iron absorption.

SUMMARY:

The Zone Diet claims to control inflammation in your body. You can use blood tests to check if you're in "the Zone." It is recommended to supplement with omega-3s and polyphenols.

Benefits of the Zone Diet

Following the Zone Diet has many benefits.

Unlike other diets, the Zone Diet does not strictly restrict any food choices.

However, it does recommend against options that are unfavorable, such as added sugar and processed foods.

This can make the Zone Diet more appealing than other diets for people who struggle with food restrictions.

The recommended food choices for the Zone Diet are quite similar to the Mediterranean Diet. The Mediterranean Diet is supported by evidence as being one of the best for your long-term health.

The Zone Diet also provides you with flexibility, since there are two methods of following the diet.

The Zone Food Block method can also help fat loss because it controls how many calories you eat per day. It is well known that controlling your calorie intake helps with weight loss .

If you want to find out how many calories you need to eat per day to maintain and lose weight, you can find out here.

SUMMARY:

The Zone Diet has many benefits linked with the favorable foods in the diet. It is flexible and may help you lose weight by helping you restrict your calorie intake.

Disadvantages of the Zone Diet

Although the Zone Diet has several benefits, it also has some disadvantages.

First, the Zone Diet makes many strong health claims that are based on the theory behind the diet.

However, there is little evidence to support that the theory produces the purported results.

For example, the Zone Diet claims to improve performance. However, a study on athletes following the diet found that, although they lost weight, they also lost endurance and were exhausted faster than others.

Reducing diet-induced inflammation to reach "the Zone" is another claim the diet makes. The Zone

Diet claims that once your blood values meet their targets, your body would be in "the Zone."

Although some research shows the diet may improve your blood values, more research is needed before researchers can say this significantly reduces inflammation in the body.

There is also little evidence that supports the Zone Diet's 40% carb, 30% protein and 30% fat ratio as the optimal ratio for fat loss and health benefits.

Another study compared the effects of a Zone-type diet that had 40% carbs, 30% protein and 30% fat to the effects of a diet that had 60% carbs, 15% protein and 25% fat.

The study did find people on a Zone-based ratio lost more weight. However, that difference could be due to higher protein intake.

Interestingly, the study also found no significant differences in blood values of sugar, fat and cholesterol between the two groups.

This does not match the claims made by the Zone Diet and could mean the improved blood values found in other studies may be due to supplementing with omega-3 and polyphenols, rather than benefits from diet alone.

SUMMARY:

The Zone Diet makes hefty health claims. However, there isn't enough evidence to support them.

Should you try the Zone Diet?

At the end of the day, choose a diet that best matches your lifestyle.

The Zone Diet could be ideal for you if you want a diet that has similar food options to the Mediterranean Diet, but provides you with clear guidelines to follow.

However, the health claims the diet makes are best taken with a grain of salt.

Although the theory behind the diet may be linked with better health outcomes, there is not enough evidence to say the diet will reduce your risk of chronic disease, slow down aging, improve physical performance or help you think faster.

If you want to try to build healthy eating habits, the Zone Diet may help get you started and help you practice portion control.

Yet what matters in the long term is basing your diet around whole and unprocessed foods — regardless of the name of the diet.

Most Diets Don't Work for Weight Loss After a Year: Here's Why

 Share on PinterestMost diets work but just temporarily. Getty Images

- A new study finds most diets lead to weight loss and lower blood pressure, but that these desired effects largely disappear after a year.

- In the study, people followed popular diets like paleo, keto, or Mediterranean. But after about a year, few kept the weight off.

- People who are interested in losing weight, and maintaining it, need a more sustainable plan than simply going on a diet.

Weight loss and weight management are two very popular topics among Americans. Just look at any Instagram feed after the holidays or right before the summer season.

While dieting does produce impressive initial results, a new international study published in The BMJ shows that most diets, regardless of which one, lead to weight loss and lower blood pressure, but these desired effects largely disappear after a year.

Approximately 45 million Americans go on a diet each year.

The study was based on the results of 121 random trials with nearly 22,000 patients. The average age was 49, and each person followed a popular named diet — like paleo, keto, or Mediterranean — or an alternative control diet — like counting macros — and reported weight loss and changes in cardiovascular risk factors.

According to the study, evidence shows that most macronutrient diets, over 6 months, result in moderate weight loss and substantial improvements in cardiovascular risk factors like blood pressure. However, after 12 months, the effect on weight reduction and improvements in cardiovascular risk factors largely disappear.

A similar study from 2018, which followed 29 long-term weight loss studies, showed that more than half of the lost weight was regained within 2 years, and by 5 years, more than 80 percent of lost weight was regained.

What this suggests is that people who are interested in losing weight, and maintaining it, need a more sustainable plan than simply going on a diet.

Why diets are short term

Typically when someone starts a diet, they see weight loss right away, especially if they're motivated and stick to that diet. But eventually, as the body loses weight, metabolism slows down and often people forget to adjust other behaviors.

"As you lose weight, your metabolism fights back against you and makes it harder to continue with that downward trend," said Sharon Zarabi, RD, CDN, CPT, bariatric program director, Lenox Hill Hospital, New York. "We need to be more in tune with what works best for us, without feeling deprived, causing us to bounce back to prior unhealthy eating styles, whether it be macros, intervals of feeding, or portion control."

How to fight back

"When people start out on a diet, they're usually very gung-ho, and it may be easier for them to meal prep or keep a fridge stocked with healthy food," said Despina Hyde-Gandhi, MS, registered dietitian at NYU Langone's Weight Management Program. "As the weeks go on, whatever behavior they changed from initially starts to come back. We have to work with patients to make a total lifestyle change, not just a diet. That's where we see a lapse in success."

What's a total lifestyle change? The recipe isn't so mysterious. In fact, it's pretty straightforward. It comes down to eating right and exercise. One of the biggest things that experts see with people looking to maintain weight is exercise. Calorie restriction is good, but to keep it off, physical activity and exercise have to increase to create lean body mass. The more lean mass a person has, the more elevated their metabolism can be.

"Doing what works for you is really important," Hyde-Gandhi added. "There's a lot of advice out there, from keto to paleo, and intermittent fasting. Some people feel great when they do these things, and some people feel lousy. You need to identify what works best for you and find balance in your meal structure."

She recommends a rule of 50-25-25, where 50 percent of each meal is vegetables, 25 percent is lean protein, and 25 percent is high fiber carbs. "If you follow that formula, weight loss aside, you'll feel well and your blood sugars will be balanced, which is helpful in maintaining your weight."

Her other recommendations for staying healthy, weight loss or not, include:

- 7 hours of sleep per night

- 64 to 80 ounces of water per day

- 150 minutes of exercise per week

"There is no one diet that works for all," said Zarabi. "It's what works best for you and is most sustainable for the long term. Any change you make to the daily food intake while lowering your total calories, will, in fact, assist in weight loss. The question is for how long."

Missing Critical Healthy Foods Also Key Reason for Diet-Related Deaths

Having a healthy diet can lead to a longer life. But it's not just about avoiding certain types of foods. It's about eating enough of the right kinds as well.

Are enough critical foods a part of your diet?

A study published in LancetTrusted Source recently reported that bad diets now kill more people in the world than smoking.

However, this trend isn't simply because of the unhealthy foods people are eating. It's also because of the critical foods people should have in their diets that they're not eating.

The study found that 11 million deaths per year across almost 200 countries could be attributable to dietary risk factors with almost more than half of those deaths attributed to lower intake of certain healthy foods.

While about 3 million deaths around the world were attributed to too much sodium, another 3 million are likely the cause of not eating enough whole grains.

Moreover, the study attributed about 2 million deaths to lack of fruit intake.

"In the past, the emphasis in the public realm, but also among health professionals, has largely been what to eliminate from our diet and the focus has been on the harmful dietary factors. However, the new science of nutrition points out that many foods that are health promoting can actually be more important or as important to include in a diet," Dr. William Li, president and medical director of The Angiogenesis Foundation and author of, "Eat to Beat Disease: The New Science of How Your Body Can Heal Itself," told Healthline.

Li explained that this doesn't mean super foods exist, but that it's more about how the body responds to food rather than the food itself.

"Health, which is what we're aiming for with diet, is not just the absence of disease, but is the result of our body's natural defense systems that are hardwired into us [and] functioning to protect our health from the time we're born until our very last breath," he said.

Activating your health defense systems with food

In his book, he discusses the following five core health defense systems and how each system is activated by certain foods.

• Angiogenesis, which is how the body grows blood vessels. Blood vessels bring oxygen and nutrients to every cell in the body.

• Regenerative system, which involves stem cells that are naturally present in our bodies.

• Microbiome, which is the healthy bacteria that lives inside our body and communicates with our immune system to help us heal faster.

• DNA, which can protect our body from the environment, such as damaging ultraviolet radiation or secondhand smoke.

• Immune system, which can fight infection and even cancer.

"It is absolutely vital for us to consume foods that help support our health defense systems," Li said. "Consuming those foods allow us to overcome the potential damage from eating unhealthy foods."

Foods to eat

Colleen D. Webb, registered dietitian nutritionist and OMG! Nutrition advisory board member, agrees with the Lancet study that most people don't eat enough whole or minimally processed fruits.

She also suggests adding more vegetables, legumes, nuts, and seeds to your diet.

"These plant foods contain necessary vitamins, minerals, fiber, and other disease-fighting chemicals we cannot get from highly processed foods or animal products," Webb told Healthline.

"Studies repeatedly show how people who eat more fruits, vegetables, and other plants live longer and better lives."

Plums

Plums are one of the more than 200 foods Li recommends in his book.

Plums are considered a stone fruit, meaning they have flesh or pulp that encloses a stone. Apricots, peaches, mangoes, and cherries are other stone fruits.

"We know that many stone fruits have [the] ability to... activate all five of those health defense systems," said Li.

Other healthful foods in Li's book include the following.

Tree nuts

Tree nuts such as walnuts, almonds, hazelnuts, cashews, and pistachios, contain a large number of polyphenols as well as omega-3 fatty acids, which are associated with a decreased risk of many cancers.

If you eat animal protein, Webb says cold-water fatty fish, such as salmon, sardines, and anchovies are also good sources of omega-3 fatty acids.

"Omega-3 fats are essential because our bodies can't make them so we must get them from food or supplements," said Webb. "Omega-3 fats help fight inflammation, stabilize mood, and support a healthy nervous system, among other benefits."

Nuts also contain a lot of dietary fiber, which feeds our gut bacteria.

"What our gut bacteria does to the fiber is that the bacteria actually digest the fiber that we don't digest," Li said. "So we chew and swallow the nut. Then our bodies absorb a lot of components of the nutritious parts of the nuts, and leave the fiber to the bacteria. The bacteria actually digest the fiber, and little pieces of the fiber that the bacteria munch on float away. Those fragments are anti-inflammatory."

Cinnamon

Cinnamon contains cinnamic acid.

Li explained this is important because, "Part of food's complexity is that they contain natural chemicals called bioactives. When we consume food [with bioactives, it] actually interacts with our human cells and also our gut bacteria."

Li said cinnamic acid is a natural chemical that is a bioactive that has anti-angiogenic effects. This means it can actually can help prune away undesirable blood vessels that might grow things like cancer.

Jasmine tea

This type of tea contains a bioactive called EGCG, which is in a family of natural compounds called catechin.

"Jasmine tea is green tea that is enhanced in terms of its flavor with jasmine flowers. So while we sometimes think of them as different teas from
a tea connoisseur's perspective, in reality jasmine tea is green tea with the scent of jasmine

flowers," Li said. "In fact, even black tea can mobilize your stem cells."

Red wine and beer

The alcohol in wine and beer does not have any health benefits.

However, the process of making red wine extracts bioactives from the skin of red grapes, and keeps it in the wine.

"[The bioactives] have been shown to be remarkable for cardiovascular health, and in small quantities for being able to even prevent cancer," Li said.

Beer is made from barley and hops. The process of making beer involves extracting a natural bioactive chemical xanthohumol from the hops.

Xanthohumol can cut off the blood supply feeding cancers and also help to mobilize stem cells that can help rebuild and regenerate the body.

"Mother Nature's incredibly clever and efficient," said Li. "Oftentimes these natural bioactive chemicals in foods have multiple job descriptions and they can activate multiple health defenses at the same time."

Nevertheless, while drinking small amounts of red wine or beer have been linked to various health benefits, the effects of alcohol can vary greatly from person to person.

Alcohol abuse and alcohol addiction have been linked to severe negative effects on both physical and mental health.

If you enjoy alcohol and don't binge, there is no compelling reason to avoid it. Just keep in mind that your cancer risk may increase — regardless of how much you are drinking.

Sourdough bread

Sourdough bread is made with bacteria called Lactobacillus reuteri, which creates the tangy flavor of the bread. Lactobacillus is bacteria found in the gut.

"Lactobacillus helps boost our immune system, helps to a accelerate our body's ability to heal a wound, and also communicates with our brain to release the social hormone oxytocin," said Li.

Although, baking the bread can kill the bacteria, Li says research has shown that remnants of the bacteria are sufficient enough to provide benefits.

Webb adds that gut health should be priority.

"Your gut digests your food and absorbs its life-supporting nutrients. Also, your gut houses much of your immune system and gut microbiome. These two work together to support a strong gut barrier, which protects you from harmful environmental factors, such as toxins and bacteria. When this barrier breaks down, we get sick," she said.

And while you add healthy foods to your diet, Webb warns that it's possible to overeat healthy foods, too.

"Be mindful of portion sizes. Stop eating before you're full. Chew your food well and eat slowly to optimize digestion," she said.